WISE CRACKS AND FUNNY BONES

FUN WITH THE CHIROPRACTOR

By

Donald McDowall

ISBN: 1-4107-6347-1 (e-book)
ISBN: 1-4107-6348-X (Paperback)

Library of Congress Control Number: 2003094704

This book is printed on acid free paper.

Printed in the United States of America
Bloomington, IN

1st Books - rev. 07/03/03

Also by Dr Donald McDowall

A Clinical Approach to Health Through Food Programming

Psychic Surgery – The Philippines Experience

Healing – Doorway to the Spiritual World

Clinical Pearls for Better Health

Http://www.chiroclinic.com.au.

CAUTION

This book is not intended to replace medical advice or to be a substitute for a physician. If you are sick or suspect you are sick, you should see a physician. If you have no sense of humour then it could already be too late.

Prevention will always be the best medicine. However, prevention can be undertaken only by the individual, and that includes humour. Laughter is the foundation of a healthy lifestyle. You have to live, so you may as well laugh .

Although this book is about humour, the author and the publisher expressly disclaim responsibility for any adverse effects arising from following the advice given in this book without appropriate medical supervision.

DEDICATION

To my wife for her tolerance of my compulsive hoarding and book collecting.

Acknowledgements

I want to thank all the patients who made me laugh.

No real names are used – to protect the innocent! However, individuals may recognise their own stories.

I also wish to thank James Homes for assisting with the editing.

Thank you to Tony Kentuck for the great cartoons.

I wish to thank Kym Bryce for her continuing devotion to the cause (and her exquisite transcription, typing and editing skills). She is also to blame for any typo's!

CONTENTS

Foreword

Some doctors think they would have the ideal practice if it were not for the patients! Others celebrate the diversity of the people who consult them. Donald McDowall is this second kind of doctor. The chiropractic doctor-patient encounter remains unique in today's health care environment because it is low-tech, high-touch, patience-centred care. Even though the touch required to deliver the spinal adjustment has such immense healing power, it remains invasive, and as humans and patients we develop little mechanisms to help us adapt to and accept this intervention.

During nearly 30 years of chiropractic practice in Australia's capital, Canberra, Donald has cared for patients of all kinds from the newborn to the nation's power-brokers. The innocence of comments made by way of a coping mechanism by patients from all walks of life reveals much of the human spirit.

Dr McDowall has captured many such comments made by his patients and this collection makes for enjoyable, thoughtful reading. This little volume tells a big story about human nature and how we see ourselves. Above all, it captures a sense of the freedom and fun that comes with the trust we extend to those who help us to heal.

Phillip Ebrall B.App.Sc.(Chiropractic), Ph.D., F.I.C.C.

Senior Lecturer in Chiropractic, RMIT University

Introduction

How do doctors cure themselves? When doctors have a problem, to whom do they go for help? The old adage "doctor, heal thyself", is often true. I pose these questions to let you know how this book began.

A few years ago I went through a lot of life changes. Some were very difficult to accept. In hindsight I now realise that it was very difficult to move on when I still clung to old ideals.

In the process of trying to understand my circumstances and what was happening in my life, I phoned my mentor Dr George Goodheart, in Detroit, Michigan, USA. George had been in Chiropractic practice for over 50 years. I figured that he would know how to solve some problems that I was still trying to work on. Being one to avoid unnecessary experiences, by trying to learn from the wisdom of others, I sought his advice.

I explained to George that I had come to a turning point in my life and really was not sure what to do next. He explained that the most important thing in these situations is to keep moving forward by being where you are appreciated and doing what you do well.

I did two things to find out how I was appreciated. The first involved my 40th birthday. I decided to have a birthday party and invite everyone I knew to come and share it with me. As well as inviting a few close friends and family, I decided to invite ALL my patients. I then gave my staff the daunting task of sending birthday party invitations to our entire mailing list. When we totalled the list, there were 14,000 names and addresses.

We sent out the invitations, organised the venue, invited entertainment and waited for the replies. We provided a phone number for RSVP. Little did I know that so many people would call at the same time. However, as well as my staff nearly going crazy from preparing the mailing list, the phones went nearly as crazy with all the RSVPs.

We had a wonderful evening of celebration!

I recommend that at least once in your life, you should find out how many people want to share a happy occasion with you. We video-taped the evening, and with all the interviews that were done, it was a wonderful lift to the spirits.

The second thing I did was to look for a way to cheer myself up on a daily basis. When I attended my patients, they would describe their problems in very colourful ways. Some of these were very novel and often made me chuckle. But as soon as the patient left, I would forget what they had said and move on to the next patient. This is necessary for a doctor, so that your mind is open and clear to listen to each patient. Over the years I had learned that listening to the patient not only reveals what the problem is, but if you listen carefully enough, very often the patient will even tell you the answer.

Dr Goodheart had often explained this in his lectures, but he had also added: "After the patient has finished talking to you, you should very carefully forget the unnecessary information". So by the time I left the consulting room, after each patient, my mind had erased the often-colourful conversations.

I decided that if I could recall these conversations from time to time, it would not only cheer me up, but also help me look at things from the patient's point of view.

Today, medical journals often discuss how important it is for doctors to do this. At first I tried writing down what the patient said after the consultation. However, I soon found out that in the process of writing, I was missing essential parts of the stories. The Dictaphone worked a lot better.

Gradually the file of stories grew into this collection.

Now and then, as I needed a little cheering up, I would pull out the file and read the stories. It became an inspiration to me that no matter how much pain people were in; they could always look on the bright side. This had healing effects as well. As people became more optimistic, began to laugh a little, and even laugh at themselves, they would relax and invariably feel better. These stories did the same for me.

As my life changed I didn't have to pick up this file as often. In fact I forgot about it for quite a number of years until a recent reorganisation of my office. In the process of sorting things out, I found this file. I showed it to a journalist friend. He suggested I have a cartoonist read it and add some sketches.

Mr Tony Kentuck happily accepted the challenge and presented me with a variety of cartoons to add to the book. I hope you enjoy his contribution as much as I do.

A chiropractor's office is a little different to a medical office. Often by the time people come to see a chiropractor they have already been to their general practitioner, a specialist, a therapist, a masseur and other health providers. They come to see us still with their pain, often having suffered for many years. They are usually frustrated, sometimes having spent hundreds and thousands of dollars trying to resolve their discomfort.

Amid all this tension and frustration we do our best to help our patients by looking at their health from a different point of view. This view empowers them with more confidence and trust.

I remember one patient saying to me that he was so frustrated with his problem and had been to so many doctors, he described my services as being *the sixth cab on the rank*! I find it sad that so many people are left for such a long time before their neighbour or another caring friend refers them for our services. Only recently has traditional medical care seen the value of chiropractic services and decided to begin the referral process. Yet in so many ways chiropractic skills have been practiced since early Egyptian times.

Manipulative techniques were the foundation for modern orthopaedics. Many specialties today would not exist had it not been for these pioneers. The sad fact is that politics often gets in the way. Egos then exaggerate the politics. In the end the only one who suffers is the patient. Instead of being quickly and efficiently directed to the services of a chiropractor, many people are misdirected, bullied and even threatened if they so much as mention the word "chiropractor" in front of their medical practitioner.

In the current climate of evidence-based medicine, chiropractic care has shone. The population is looking for results, not politics. It is looking for care and communication.

So you see, in this environment the following stories have bubbled to the surface. I have credited no one individually for their stories, but wish to thank all those patients who contributed to this book. They will know who they are when they read the stories.

Humour is good for the soul and laughing at our own problems is often an essential part of the healing process. Not taking ourselves too seriously is an adage with great healing power. Hopefully, I have achieved that goal in this collection.

Enjoy!

Donald A. McDowall, DC, DIBAK

June 2003

Chapter One

A patient commented after having her treatment, "Doctor every time I finish with you I feel like a potato chip". I said, "Why do you say that?" She said, "I feel all scrunched up."

Avoiding a problem is better than prevention and prevention is better than cure.

A patient explained about the pain that she was getting when she was sleeping. She said, "Doctor, I want to know why I'm no good in bed?" How do you answer a question like that?

A patient tried to describe the different noises she felt in her spine. She said to me, "Doctor can you tell me why I bang and crunch so much?"

A patient explained, "Doctor my neck is off today, do you think you can put it back in place for me?"

A patient limped in to the office bent dramatically to the right and said, "Doctor I feel just like an old farmer checking his fences on a cold morning."

A patient attended for a check-up and after treatment explained to me, "You know Doctor, every time you treat me like this and make me turn from side to side and up and down, I feel just like I have been rotisseried. I hope you don't think I'm an old chook." I said to her, "No, I will treat you as gentle as a lamb."

After I recommended exercises for a low back condition, a patient explained to me, "Doctor the only exercise I get is jumping to conclusions."

A patient asked me if I had heard about the lady who attended the psychiatrist. I said "No". He said she explained to the psychiatrist that she wasn't sure whether she was a wigwam or a tepee. The psychiatrist looked at her and said, "Don't worry, I think that your problem is that you are too tense *[two tents]*."

After treating a patient I asked how his wife was. He said she was feeling much better after she had been treated and was now playing lawn bowls. As was customary with bowls, often the prizes are frozen chickens. I said to him, "Did she win any chickens today?" He looked at me and said, "No, but there were plenty of old white leghorns out there."

A woman patient explained to me that things weren't always what they seem in life. She said that a friend told her about a nurse who, while working in a hospital, met an old man in his seventies. Every morning he would give her a little plastic bag of almonds. She would take them and share them with her friends, until one day they felt quite guilty about eating his food. They thought that perhaps his relatives were expecting him to eat them and that it wasn't right for them to. So one morning the nurse said to the old man, "Thank you very much for the almonds, but we really don't think that we should take them from you any more, you need them more than we do." The old man looked at her, smiled gently, and said to her, "That's all right dear, I only like the chocolate covering on the outside."

A woman attending with her young child said, "We were preparing to come and see you this morning and my young son said to me, 'Mummy, are we going to the chiropractor today?' I said yes. He said, 'Oh good, can I have a turn too?" Somewhat surprised she said, "Usually you don't ask like this." He said, "No, but today I want to have a 'crick-crack front and back'."

A selfish child's attitude towards a parent is: I deserve what I want. You're responsible for me. Therefore you suffer when you fill my needs.

A patient complained of low back pain and said, "Doctor I think I am wearing out, do you think that's normal for my age?" I looked at her and said, "I don't think you need to call it 'wearing out', just maturing would be adequate."

With back pain, the truth of the discomfort always shows a few days after the reality of the injury.

Chapter Two

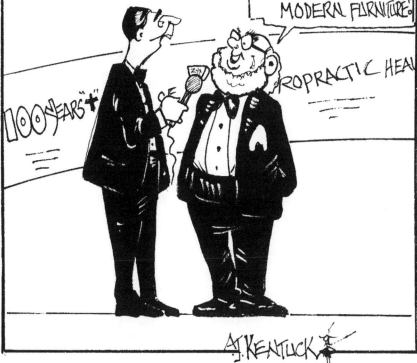

A patient attempting to describe her pain, commented, "Doctor take it easy with me today, I feel tender all over, even worse than a good steak."

A patient with a sore throat said, "Doctor I have a prickly throat. It feels like razor rash. What causes that?"

A new patient was getting ready for x-ray examination. I explained that she should take all her clothes off except her panties and put the gown on so that it opened at the back. She smiled, turned around, looked at me and said, "And do you do the same Doctor?"

A patient's opening comments to me were "Doctor I have a kangaroo back." I said, "What is a kangaroo back?" She said, "It keeps jumping out of place all the time. Can you tell me what to do with it?"

A patient so distressed with her pain and discomfort commented, "Doctor I feel so bad, do you think I could go back where I came from?" She then said, "It would probably be all right, but I think the warranty has expired and he probably wouldn't take me."

A patient commented, "Doctor I just feel out of touch with everything. I am so busy running around I can't feel a thing."

A patient with Meniere's disease (vertigo) said to me "Doctor, I feel like Dick Van Dyke." I said, "Why is that?" She said, "I fall over at the drop of a hat."

A patient attended who seemed nervous and somewhat distressed. As I was treating her I said, "What seems to be the problem?" She explained, "Well, chiropractors hurt nearly as much as the dentist." I asked, "Why do you feel that way? Have you had a bad experience with a dentist?" She looked at me and said, "Yes, dentists lie through their teeth and I haven't yet worked out how chiropractors do it."

A patient so excited about her progress said, "You know Doctor, I really feel better when I'm better, in fact everyone feels better when I'm better." I said, "Thank you, I even feel better when everyone else feels you're as better as you think you are. In fact, you are better."

After a hip adjustment the patient commented, "Doctor if you keep pulling my leg like that, I'm going to end up walking around cross-legged. I'm bad enough as it is, walking around in circles all day."

A patient concerned about the re-occurring problems in her neck explained to me one day, "You know Doctor, I think this neck is going to be the death of me. If only someone could chop it out I think I would be all right." I said to her, "Head transplants are hard to get! No one wants to donate a good one."

During a patient's second visit I asked, "How are you feeling today?" She explained, "I have this terrible pain across my shoulders and it's just been annoying me all day." Somewhat set back I asked her, "What about the headache you had yesterday, and the low back pain?" "Oh," she said, "those are gone, it's just this terrible pain across my shoulders." Perceiving I must have been a little concerned about my lack of success with her, she looked at me and said, "Don't worry Doctor, two out of three isn't bad, you can get this one better for next time."

A patient described the pain that she felt in her hips, she said, "Doctor my hip keeps going on and off, on and off, on and off, and now I don't know what to do with it or where to put it."

A patient whose husband I had been helping for muscle weakness in the arms, said to me, "My husband feels so much better now. Now when he hugs and squeezes me he feels like he means it."

A patient was concerned about the noises in her neck and said to me, "Doctor I think the only way to get rid of the noise is for you to put a grease nipple on either side of my neck and then I can fix it myself."

Chapter Three

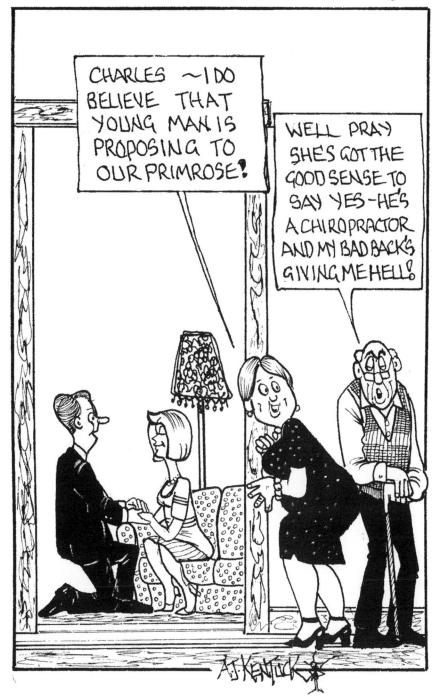

Donald McDowall

A patient obviously in need of treatment exclaimed, "I'm all dragged out today. I just knew I needed a good going over. Do you think you can give me one?"

As I was giving instructions to a patient for positioning for her adjustments, I could see she was becoming irritable and edgy. I asked her what seemed to be the problem and she said, "Doctor you speak so softly. I have a hearing disability and I do wish you would stop whispering in my ear, you have to treat me differently than other women, you've got to shout to get my attention!"

Some people you can talk to, to get their attention. Other people you have to talk at.

After stimulating some acupressure reflexes on a patient that were quite tender, she commented, "You're not very gentle Doctor. You wouldn't make a very good woman."

A patient commented after treatment, "Doctor every time I have my treatment with you I feel like I am a rabbit." I said, "Why is that?" She answered, "It's just like I have been through a hedge."

A patient concerned about her shoulder posture asked, "Doctor do you think I am getting better? My clothes don't seem to fall off me any more?"

A patient feeling somewhat concerned about the discomfort and nerve pain she was feeling in the lower calf area of her leg said, "Doctor I have this feeling of hot oil running down the side of my leg, that gradually intensifies and becomes very irritable. Where do you think it's coming from?" And then with a slight grin she said, "Do you think my 'diff' is leaking?"

While waiting for me in the treatment room, a patient commented that she saw the empty chain hanging from my ceiling and said, "I was wondering what that chain was for. Did the pot plant die or is that where you hang the difficult ones?"

A patient tried to describe the fatigue and discomfort he felt sporting two black eyes and a big bump in the middle of his forehead after catching a cricket ball with his head. His comment was, "I think I am a gardener's delight today; they nearly had to bury me, I am about as seedy as they come at the moment."

After reflecting on her previous treatment, a patient commented, "Doctor please be gentle with me today, I feel like a dry biscuit. When you crunch me I don't want to crumble all over."

A patient having difficulty with her co-ordination said, "Doctor I have all this trouble. I just keep getting all mixed up between my arms and legs. What can I do?"

A patient had been relaxing on the treatment table. As I entered the room she said, "Doctor you need some nice soft lighting in these rooms for people like me."

A patient was attempting to describe the discomfort she felt in her stomach in a particular bending posture: "When I am doing my yoga exercise, I have to bend my arms between my legs and huff and puff at the same time. Why do I feel so uncomfortable?"

A patient wanted me to help her feet and commented, "Doctor will you try and see how far you can pull my feet off my ankles today, please."

A patient was intrigued about the knee jerk neurological tests that I was doing. After watching her leg kick out several times she looked at me and said, "Doctor you're the only person who can get such a big rise out of me."

A patient explained that she had low back pain during intercourse. After examination I said to her that she would need to have a rest for a few days until her back healed. She said, "In that case, I will need to have a note for my husband!"

Chapter Four

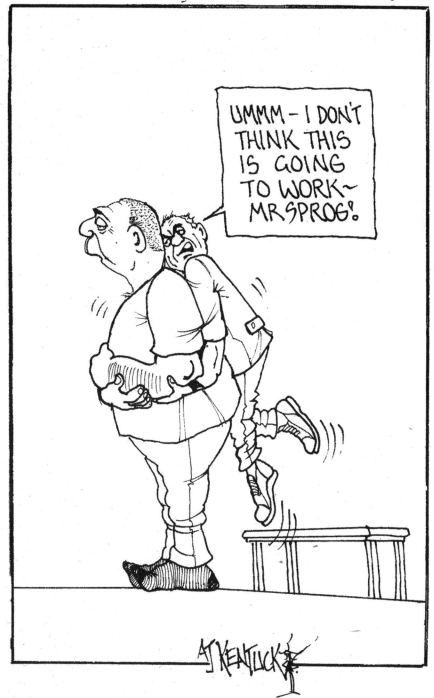

Donald McDowall

A pregnant patient attended with low back pain. After treating some acupressure reflexes she commented, "What are you trying to do Doctor, give me practice for coping with labour pain?"

A patient was attempting to describe discomfort he was feeling and the frustration of trying to keep his back in good shape. The anatomical considerations of his comment were quite interesting: "Doctor I feel like my back is falling apart around my ears."

A patient explained she felt that her body was "all compressed together". "Doctor, I feel like my tailbone is sitting under my chin."

As a patient was making her return appointment I commented to the receptionist, "I think this patient would like to have an early morning appointment probably around 10am." The patient looked at me, smiled and said, "Yes, a gentle 10am."

A patient explained that she was having trouble sleeping and commented, "Doctor I find that I just can't sleep at night. I think it's because I get so excited." I was unsure about asking her what was the cause of her excitement. She then explained that she was preparing for an overseas holiday and was excited in anticipation.

A patient concerned about her condition explained, "Doctor I feel like a runaway truck going downhill, and going downhill at a great rate!"

A patient happy with her progress remarked, "Doctor all I've got left is my thumbs." Somewhat taken aback, considering that her initial complaints were to do with her neck and low back, I asked what she meant. She said, "I'm all thumbs today. Everything else feels so good that all I can think about is the old arthritic problems in my thumbs."

A patient whose back was so sore that he had to keep moving around all the time and couldn't stand still commented, "Doctor I don't think they'd employ me as a 'Stop and Go' man." I asked, "What do you mean a 'Stop and Go' man?" He answered, "You know, those road workers who have to stand in one spot all day turning the signs around that say Stop and Go. I'd be so fidgety I wouldn't be able to concentrate on the sign and people wouldn't know whether they were coming or going."

A patient concerned about losing her hair said, "Doctor my hair just keeps falling out. I feel like a chicken in the middle of moulting season."

A patient suffering from a painful head exclaimed, "Doctor are you good with soreheads?"

A patient concerned about his frequency of visits commented, "Doctor I'm breaking my back to earn money to pay you to help my back."

A patient said, "Doctor I feel like a drug addict. I need a fix for my neck this morning."

I was explaining to a patient how to maintain correct posture to reduce pain in her arms and told her that she had to keep her chin tucked in all the time. She said, "Is this what my husband means when he says I need to pull my head in?"

An older patient trying to describe how well she felt explained, "Doctor I just feel so good. I know I am going to die a well women!"

A patient explained how relaxed she was after having her adjustments. She said, "I was so relaxed I even put the sugar in my mother's fridge."

A patient with headaches after attending a Christmas party explained that she didn't feel the season of good will was doing her as much good as it should. "In fact," she said, "I think it's really the season of good will and poor judgement!"

Life is always good. Sometimes we just expect more than we deserve.

Chapter Five

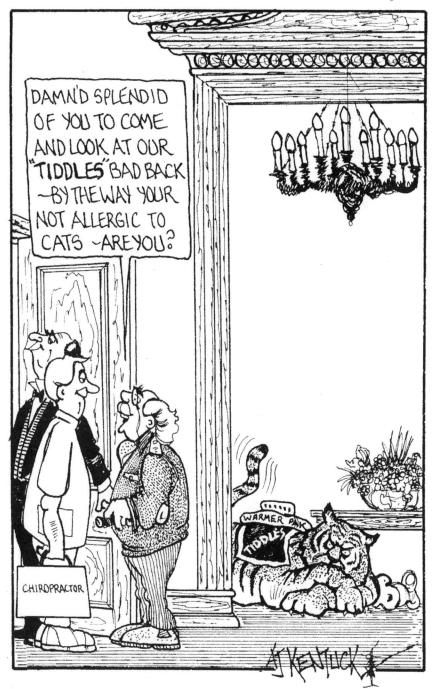

25

Donald McDowall

A patient explained "Doctor I have these kinky joints. What can I do with them?"

After trying a special neck pillow to help his problem, a patient said, "Doctor that new pillow you gave me is just driving me around the twist. All I do is toss and turn all night."

After hearing all the noises in her neck from the treatment, the patient commented, "You know Doctor, my young son doesn't refer to you as a chiropractor. He calls you the crick-cracktor."

A young lady patient had a business involving T-shirt designs. After getting her adjustment one day she said, "Doctor I have designed this chiropractic T-shirt. I was wondering if you would like to order them for your patients?" I asked, "Do you have one for me to look at?" She said, "Yes" and then took off her shirt revealing a T-shirt underneath which said "My chiropractor keeps me loose." While appreciating her enthusiasm for marketing the product, I had to explain to her that I wasn't sure that I could support her sharing that opportunity with all my patients.

A patient somewhat concerned about the sore neck she had explained, "Doctor my neck is stuck. I think it needs a good swivelling."

A patient was somewhat hesitant about the discomfort she might experience with the adjustments. She said, "Doctor are these walls thick enough so that if I make a lot of noise nobody will hear me?" I replied, "Yes, they are soundproof, you can scream as loud as you like." She said, "Oh no, you don't have to worry about that, I'll scream softly and that way I won't have to holler harder."

A patient tried to describe the discomfort he had with his back condition. He said, "Doctor I have difficulty bending over shaving in the morning unless I put my shoes on. If I put my shoes on then I find I can bend over and wash my face after I have shaved, but then after I have shaved I've got to take my shoes off to put my pants on and when I bend over to put my pants on, my back gets sore again and I have trouble putting my shoes on. What I would really like to do is understand how I can bend over and wash my face after shaving, before I put my shoes on, but after I put my pants on so that my back doesn't hurt. Do you think you can help me?"

Donald McDowall

A patient concerned about the discomfort he was feeling said, "Doctor when I wake up in the morning, I wake up with a limp and it just doesn't go away until I warm up. Do you think you can help me?" I asked, "What part of your body gets the limp?" He replied, "My ankle, of course."

A patient had low back pain during the Christmas holiday season. I asked her how her back injury occurred. She explained, "I think I was carrying too much alcohol." I said, "That doesn't seem unusual at Christmas time, a lot of people seem to do that." She said, "Yes, but I couldn't even enjoy it. I was carrying it by the box and loading it on to the shelf in my father's store."

A little boy attended my Clinic for the first time in quite a lot of distress. I asked his mother why he was crying. She said that he was quite happy when he left home and she explained that he was going to the chiropractor. When they arrived at the Clinic, however, he was quite disillusioned and began to cry. She said, "I asked him why he was crying and he said, 'Mummy this isn't even Egypt'." The little boy's dad was in the public service, routinely travelled to foreign countries and when his mother mentioned that he was going to see "the chiropractor" he thought he was going to Cairo, to see the doctor and was looking forward to going to Egypt.

A patient so happy with the treatment he'd received for his neck pain exclaimed that he was as happy as a dog with two tails.

A patient was attempting to explain how his doctor had diagnosed his spinal condition. He said the doctor told him it was a case of genital spondylosis. I was somewhat surprised. I said: "You mean congenital spondylosis?" He said: "Yes."

Chapter Six

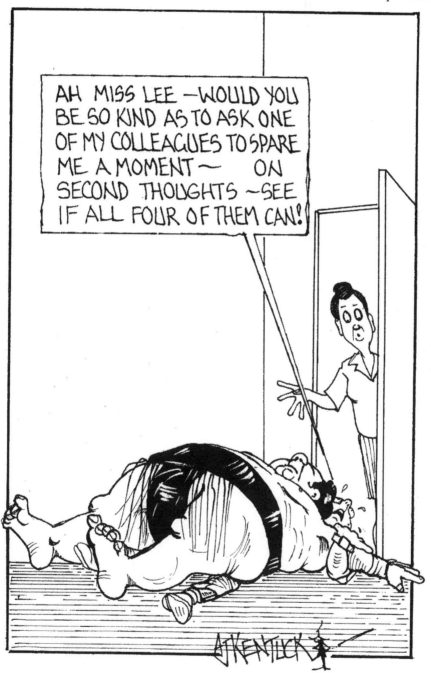

A patient, an old farmer, came in one day and explained that he had finally worked out why he has headaches. He said that when he was a child his father used to always tell him how good a hit under the ear was for him when he was disobedient. This old patient told me that he never believed it until he came to the chiropractor. He then went on to explain that had his father hit him under both the right and left ear when he was a child, instead of just under the one side, it might have evened him up and prevented his headaches in later years.

A patient was complaining about the pain in her knees when she was walking. I explained to her that the knees had become like rusty hinges and even though I couldn't give her new knees, the body would repair the joint surface and the rust would start to go away. She said, "Is that like the difference between the new tyre and a retread?"

A patient was explaining to me how she felt old at the age of 52. I said to her, but you're just a spring chicken. And she said, "No, I'm a sprung chicken."

A patient attended asking for help in the right upper thigh and buttock area. She explained that the pain occurred after she had been playing tennis. After examination I explained to her that I felt she had strained some muscles in her buttock. She said to me that she understood that tennis players sometimes got tennis elbow and is it possible that this could be what is called a "tennis bum"?

A patient explained that she had sore arms. I examined her and found a lot of soft tissue inflammation in the upper shoulder and neck areas. I asked her what she thought caused the problem. She explained that she had been aerial decorating. I said, "Aerial decorating? I don't think I've ever heard of that." She said, "That's when you throw everything on top of the refrigerator and cupboards before your baby gets to it, like garbage lids, plates, etc."

A patient explained that he had been involved in an accident earlier in his life, but that it had caused no significant problem. He had run into a cow with his motorcycle. The ambulance had taken him to the local hospital to be treated for grazing.

A patient arrived explaining that her back was painful and she felt that it was out of plumb. After I had examined her she looked me straight in the eye and said, "Do you think you can make it as good as apples?"

Chapter Seven

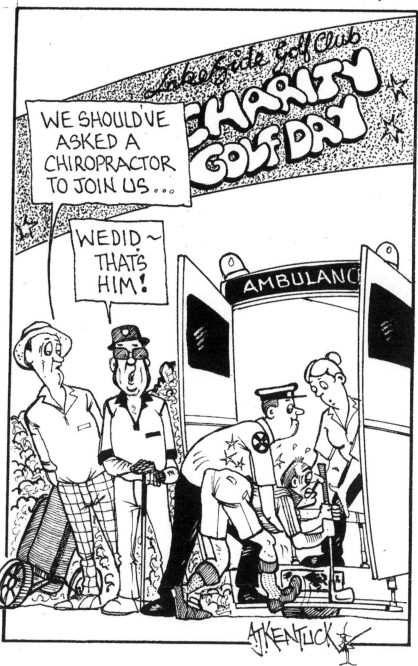

A patient explained to me that when visiting the butcher, he had answered the phone half way through serving her and started laughing. She enquired as to what was so funny. He explained that the lady had ordered 50¢ worth of meat for her cat and had just called up to cancel the order. She had said that her cat had just caught a mouse and she wouldn't need the meat today, thank you.

A patient wanted me to treat her son. She explained that he was 6'4" and growing like a mushroom. She said, "I think he has trouble keeping up with himself."

A male patient attended with low back pain that had given him trouble for some years. A man in his mid-60's, he responded well to treatment and came to the stage where I was ready to dismiss him or extend his visits further. I suggested that perhaps I could check him in about a month, but he said that he would prefer to see me in a week and I thought he still had some insecurity about his progress. I followed up and checked him the next week and gave him a minor adjustment. The patient then asked if he could see me in another week, he still felt a month was too long. At this stage I was getting a little suspicious because it is not usual to get requests for more frequent treatments, usually patients request treatments at wider intervals.

So I asked him why he wanted to see me so often. He said that he didn't want to chance not feeling well again. I said that his back had responded well and I didn't really suspect that. He said, "Well Doctor, I'm not sure how to tell you this, but since you've been giving me an adjustment my sex life has returned after being away for a number of years." He explained that he could now have an erection, whereas before he was unable to. He said that he didn't want to risk losing that and it was more important for him to have his adjustments regularly for that purpose rather than to risk losing his manhood. To this day, some five years later, he still comes regularly, but I have been able to extend his visits to three- or four-month intervals and he maintains an active sex life now in his late 70's.

A patient asked me one morning if she could have some illustrations of the spine. She said that she was giving a talk in her science class and wanted to be able to explain what spinal deviants were. I then wondered if the title "chiropractor" was adequate for someone who helped to correct spinal deviants!

A patient was telling me about her school reunion and explained that after 25 years one of her old class friends commented that she looked so good, she looked just like Greta Garbo. My patient looked me square in the eye and said "You

37

know I didn't know whether to take that as a compliment or not. Greta Garbo has been in the grave for 10 years."

A patient explained that every time she gets her treatment, the tension goes and she feels like a wet rag when she leaves.

Chapter Eight

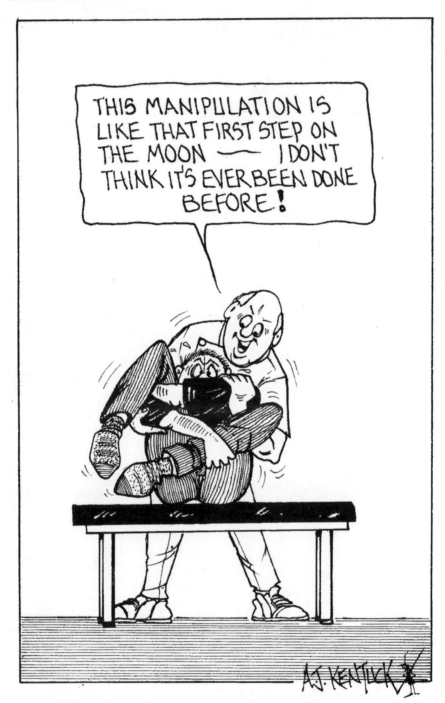

A patient presented with low back pain. She was also pregnant with twins. After treating her I said, "Well will you be doing that again?" She said, "No, I'll definitely be thinking twice."

A patient with low back pain explained, "My back was so bad this morning, my husband couldn't even put my stockings on."

A patient presented explaining that she heard that one of her friends had received good results with an adjustment and was able to get pregnant and have a baby. She then asked, "Do you think you could do the opposite adjustment, so I don't have to take contraceptives?"

A patient explained that her symptoms were so painful that some days she felt bad and other days she felt real bad. She said that she was starting to feel like Mae West.

A patient presented with low back pain and explained that he was standing in the doorway when his young son came charging through it and used him as a brake. The patient went on to say; "Now I think my linings are shot."

A patient explained that her riding instructor wanted her back to have more flexibility during her horse-riding lessons. She said, "Doctor do you think you can make my back looser? I would like to be a loose woman while I am riding."

A patient said, "Doctor I am as stiff as a board, do you think I am ready for the 'pine box'?"

A patient presented with severe neck pain and shoulder discomfort, and said to me, "Doctor I have this neck pain that just won't go away. Do you think it's possible that I'm carrying the world on my neck, and I just don't give it a chance to get down to my shoulders?"

A patient with acute low back pain explained, "Doctor my back is so sore I just can't turn over." She said with some humour in her voice, "I wouldn't make a very good rotisserie, let alone a tender chicken."

A patient presented with pain when turning and said to me, "Doctor I get so confused when you ask me to turn from left to right, I don't know which side is which. How can I be this lost and not even be away from home?"

A patient was explaining her difficulty in understanding her problem. She said, "Doctor I feel like a jigsaw puzzle. Do you think if you put me in a bag and shake me up and down I will come back together better than I am?"

A patient complained of being sore all over. She said, "Doctor do you think I am really the total pain that my husband thinks I am?"

Chapter Nine

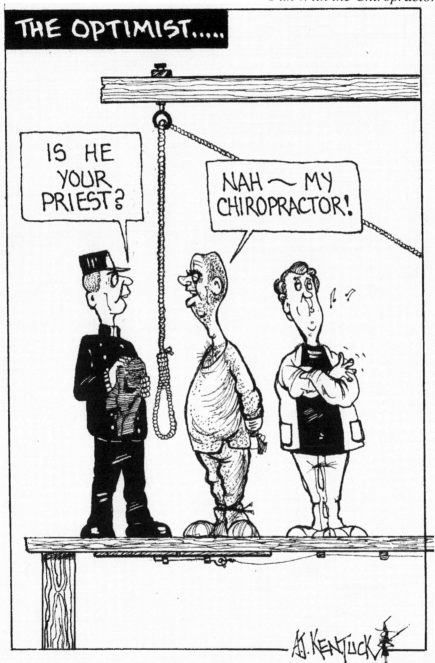

Isn't it interesting that some people have trouble keeping up with their age?

A patient was telling me that she couldn't understand why whenever something went wrong her husband always referred to the particular object that was giving him the trouble as "she". So one day she asked him and said, "Why do you refer to everything that gives you trouble as if it's a woman?" He looked her straight in the eye and said, "Because I feel like I am being nagged!"

Sometimes during treatment a little pain in the present may be worth a lot of relief in the future.

A patient explained that she felt that she was leaning over to the side and felt a little bit crooked. Her comment was, "Do you think that you can straighten me out before I turn into a politician?"

After releasing a pressure point on a patient's shoulder she commented, "That's what Mr Spock does in 'Star Trek' and people collapse when he does that." My comment was, "We do the reverse. It seems to help."

A patient asked me, "Doctor is *erection* an important part of posture?"

A patient presented with a sinus condition explaining that she had had difficulty smelling for many years and asked if I could help. She said her husband was complaining that he was the only one that could tell when the baby had a dirty nappy and of course was the one, then, that had to change it.

A nurse complained of pain in her arm and hand when taking blood pressure readings. She said, "I think I've got cuff-puffers elbow."

A patient was describing how painful her low back was and wondered if I understood what she was trying to say. I explained to her that a low back sprain is just like a sprained ankle, you have to care for it with cold/wet packs and just be careful with it. She said to me, "It might look like a sprained ankle to you, but that's not what I sit on all day."

After reviewing a slim patient's x-rays and seeing his interest in the bone structure that I was illustrating, his young daughter politely remarked, "Dad, does this really mean that you are the bag of bones that Mum says you are?"

A patient attended with acute low back pain after she had tripped. Her first comment upon seeing me was, "Doctor I think I fell for you today."

A bookkeeper presented with joint pain and made the comment, "Doctor I work with figures all day, I was wondering if you could help me with mine now?"

A patient presented in an *antalgic* (bent-over) position and expressed her concerns to me by saying, "Doctor I think my inclinations are all wrong."

A patient attended with a strained wrist. I enquired as to how this injury occurred. She explained, "My dog took me for a walk and I just couldn't keep up."

A patient explained, "Doctor my neck and back are a bit dippy. I am feeling like a roller coaster, do you think you can help?"

A patient presented suffering from hot flushes and said, "Doctor I feel like nothing on earth. Do you think this is what they call the twilight zone?"

A patient feeling some discomfort from a deep massage treatment commented, "It feels just like you're using a drill." I politely smiled at him and asked, "Do I bore you?" He said, "No, but every *bit* hurts."

It's not the worry of stress that causes the problems in people, but the stress of worry that creates the most complications.

Chapter Ten

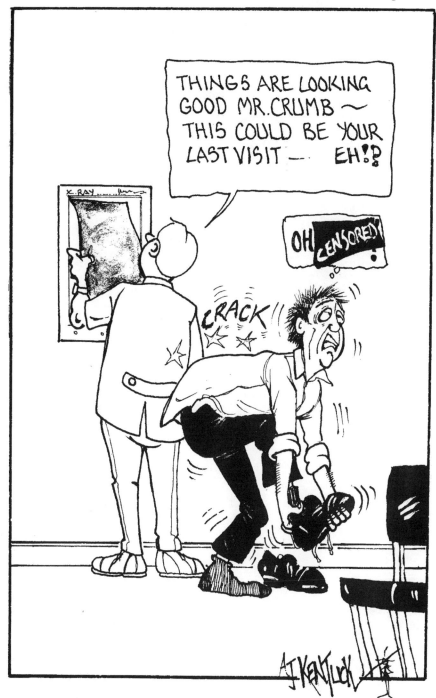

A patient said, "Doctor I don't know how you're going to work with me, I'm so bony that every time I do sit ups I rub the skin off my bottom."

After looking at a neurological chart on the wall of my office, a patient told me about the discomforts she felt and said, "I think my sympathetic nervous system has gone out in sympathy with my shoulder."

A patient suffering from a painful neck said, "Doctor I am having so much pain in my neck, I have come to put my body in your hands."

A patient was commenting on how terrible it was that people become addicted to prescribed drugs. She was discussing tranquillisers and how critical they were in causing so many addictive problems. I said to her, "Yes it's just like with chocolate, only chocolate isn't even on prescription." With some alarm she exclaimed, "Goodness, don't criticise chocolate, that's the one habit that I enjoy."

In practice you know you're on time when the patients start complaining about not having to wait.

A patient attended with her back bent and in pain. She was very concerned that she couldn't straighten up. She said that she was flying out of town the next day and was concerned that her tilted posture may upset the balance of the aeroplane and cause it to crash. She asked, "Can you straighten me up and save the lives of all the other people on the aeroplane?"

A patient attempted to describe pain in her upper back. She said, "Doctor, I get this pain right where my wings are." Her husband, who was sitting next to her in the room, explained "Yes, her wings are not in the same place as her horns." I looked at her and said, "It's good to see a person who is so optimistic about their direction in life."

While I was taking a patient to the treatment room, he looked in and said, "Ah, I get cell block no. 3 today, do I Doctor?" I asked him why he called it a "cell block" and he said, "I think it's because of all the torture I have to go through to get better."

A woman receiving treatment and advice for a dietary program, explained to me "Another doctor gave me a vegetarian diet to follow, but I think I will have to stop." When I asked her why, she explained, "I find that when I eat that way I start leaning over towards the sun. The last thing I want to do is wilt late at night."

A patient complaining of diarrhoea explained to me, "Doctor, I've been on this whole-grain diet for a number of weeks now, but I think I have become 'bran-washed'."

Chapter Eleven

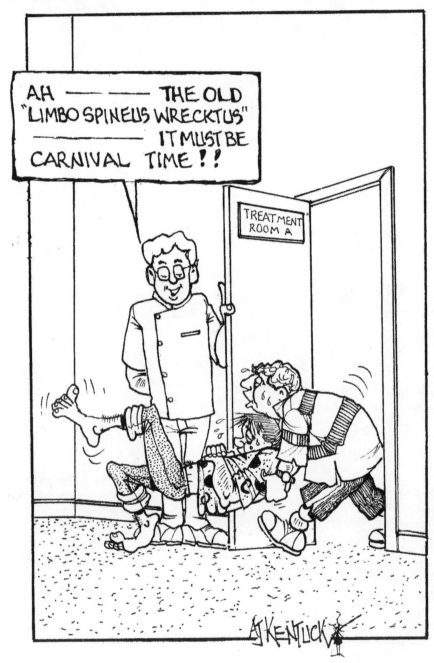

While examining a patient, she apologised for the ladder in her stocking. I told her not to worry, I didn't really take notice. She said she was very sorry, but her boyfriend was a fireman. I said that it was just such a small ladder. She said, "Yes, he didn't have to climb so high on this one." She was 68.

A young patient complained of headaches. Her mother explained that while she was playing netball, the ball had hit her right in the ear and knocked her over. The girl looked up at me and said, "Yes, it's pretty hard to hold on to a ball with your ear. I had to let it drop."

A patient attended for advice about food. I was discussing the various aspects of different types of food to her. She explained that when she was a young girl her mother made a special soup called "False" soup. When I asked her what "False" soup was, she explained, "That's soup that my father use to always complain about because it had no meat in it."

A patient with low back pain said, "Doctor, my back feels like Tarzan's Grip". When I asked her why, she said, "Because it's all glued up."

A patient explained that she had hurt her back when she fell into a hole while in the park. I tried to console her that the damage wasn't too serious. She looked at me and said, "Yes, but it very nearly could have been. I managed to crawl out of the hole before they started to throw the dirt over the top."

A patient complaining of low back pain explained, "Doctor I feel like I've been put in a sugar bag and hit with a stick."

A patient concerned about the discomfort with her adjustment, said to me "Doctor, you'll have to adjust me quickly, right between my tension and anxiety, and there probably won't be much room in between."

A patient attempting to describe pain in her low abdomen said, "Doctor, I get this pain over the full bikini area." I asked, "What do you mean by that?" She said, "If you have a very small bikini on, it covers the whole area that the bikini covers."

While waiting for me in the treatment room, a patient tried to keep himself occupied. When I opened the door he was tapping his knees with the reflex hammer. When he saw me notice what he was doing, he looked up and said, "It's all right Doctor, I'm only testing my *reflection*."

A patient explained to me that she had been at work all day and from the beginning of the day until the end, all people could do was jump on her. She said, "I think it has given me a sore back and hips. Do you think you can help me?" I said, "Yes, but you'll have to tell your friends that they won't be allowed to jump on you for at least three days after the treatment."

A mother attended as a patient with her young child. As the child became noisy I gave him a wooden tongue depressor to play with. After playing with it for a while, he looked up at me and said, "Doctor what do you do with the ice creams that come off these?"

After having good results with her adjustment, a patient said, "You know Doctor, when I first came here I had great difficulty sleeping, but with the success of your treatment I now feel confident that I can sleep anywhere."

A patient commented, "You know Doctor, every time I finish with you I feel like a used toothpaste tube."

A patient was having trouble describing all the different symptoms that she had, and while getting a little frustrated doing this, looked at me and said, "Well I think I can put it down to this, Doctor, what I've done is come to give you experience." I looked at her and said, "Just what I need, a patient who feels her doctor needs more experience. Thank you for the opportunity."

A patient attended with a sprained back and while taking her history, I asked her to explain what she felt caused it. She said, "Well last night I was dreaming that my husband ran off with another woman. I finally caught him and in the process of beating him to a pulp, I woke up and my back was sore." I said, "How did your husband feel?" She said, "I haven't even started on him yet, but he went without breakfast, and I was still mad at him in the evening." I said, "Did you explain to him why you were mad at him." When she answered that she had, I said, "What did he say?" She said, "He said 'Well perhaps I'll have to find somebody so I can justify the way I'm being treated.'" Then she said, "You know what the worst thing about the whole dream was? That cheap little floozy was only 18 years old and here I am, 46."

A rural patient explained, "Doctor I have pain in my feet, they're sore all the time and I'm having difficulty walking. Can you tell me if humans get *founder*" (Founder is a hoof disease of horses.)

A patient commented, "Doctor if you find nothing to do on me today, I'll pay you double."

A patient said, "Doctor, today I'm a sore for sight eyes."

A patient said, "I'm all yours Doctor. Do what you want. Start at the bottom and work to the top and tell me when you've finished."

Chapter Twelve

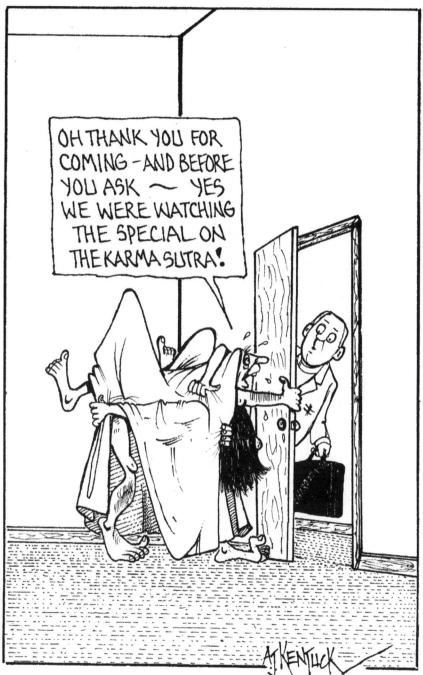

Donald McDowall

A patient attended with low back pain. I asked him if he had a medical opinion about his condition. He explained, "Yes, the doctor told me that my back was the back of a degenerate and there was nothing much he could do about it." He went on to explain, "But I don't care, because the doctor who told me that died two months ago. So now I want a new opinion."

A patient attending first thing on a winter morning and exclaimed, "Doctor your hands are so cold, I've never had you with cold hands before. Don't you dare warm them up on me!"

The trust in a relationship is directly proportional to the time spent together.

A patient attended with low back pain and stiffness. I commented, "John, I have treated you today and you were stiff in the neck, mid-back and low-back areas." He looked at me and said, "Doctor, I am just stiff all over. I even shit stiff!"

Children's enthusiasm to communicate is directly proportional to your lack of interest in listening to them.

You can't help some people and some people can't help themselves.

Life is a constant momentum of opportunities that are constructive or destructive, depending on your choice.

What is the difference between trust and respect? One can respect everyone, but trust only a few. The reason? Everyone has different priorities and the people you trust may not have the same priorities as you, yet you can respect them.

The best teacher in life is often you. The best lessons are often those you have to learn from your own experience.

People can't experience your feelings unless they have experienced what you have.

A female patient explained that when she got up that morning her husband turned over, looked at her and said, "Well dear, how do you feel today? Do you have a headache, a backache or are you just a pain in the neck?" She then said, "So I thought I'd better come and see you and find out if I am a serious problem."

A patient explained that since she had been injured the only parts of her body that worked properly were her mouth and her foot. Her daughter suggested that seeing she can't work in her old job as a teacher, that perhaps she should find a new job as a foot and mouth artist!

A patient explained to me, "Doctor I think I've just had an experience that you will probably call a constructive accident." I asked her why she said "constructive accident". She said, "Well I had this pain in my back that was very uncomfortable and as I was getting in the car to come and see you I slipped on a gravel surface, landed on my hip, felt a click in my back and now my back feels good." After examination I could not find any evidence of injury and confirmed that it was not in her imagination and that a constructive accident being a novel term, was probably also accurate in her case.

A patient explained that he had "aeroplane syndrome". When I asked him what "aeroplane syndrome" was, he said, "That's the sort of stiff neck you get from sitting in an aeroplane seat for a long time."

A patient with a sore neck explained, "Doctor I'm having trouble sighting my balls, my neck gets so sore. Do you think you can help?" I looked at him strangely and said, "How does your neck get sore sighting balls?" He said, "I'm a golfer and when I take a swing I can't look up to see where my ball goes."

A patient in her late 70's, with low back pain, said to me, "My doctor calls it a 'romantic back'." I said, "A 'romantic back'?" She said, "Yes, he thinks it's in the family." I said, "You mean RHEUMATIC." She said, "Yes, that's what I mean."

An Irish patient told me that his house nearly flooded and burnt down at the same time when his washing machine caught on fire.

Chapter Thirteen

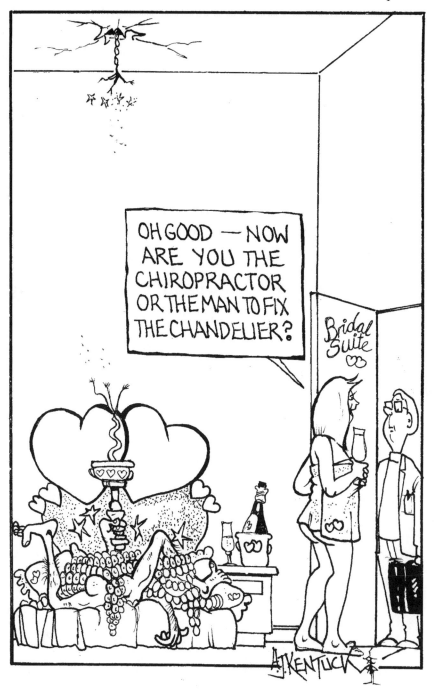

A woman's ability to change is directly proportional to a man's ability to provide.

There are two ways to do things, the wrong way and your wife's way.

We do what tradition expects us to do, or we do what we enjoy doing. The secret to getting along with everybody is to enjoy doing what tradition expects us to do.

In the course of consultation I asked a patient how he was. He responded, "Not so good today Doctor. I think I'm suffering from the old-age complaint." When I asked him what he meant by that, he looked at me and said, "Nothing works when I want it to any more."

A young male patient explained that his neck was very sore. I asked him what happened, how did he cause the problem. He said, "Well you won't believe this Doctor, but I was looking under my arm to see if I had used enough deodorant and my neck clicked and got stuck!"

Patient explained that he had liquorice back. When I asked what that was, he explained, "That's the back that you get when you have liquorice diarrhoea, sitting on the toilet and then you strain your back so bad that you can't get up again. I think they should have warning labels on bags of liquorice like they have on cigarettes, such as: 'warning, this liquorice may give you such severe diarrhoea that you will hurt your back.'" Fortunately we were able to help him find a cure for his problem.

A patient asked me to explain the reason for her child's bleeding nose. I said to her, "The blood vessels in the nose are very fragile and with changes in temperature or humidity they can overstretch and bleed very quickly." I then went on to explain that it was similar with the uterus; that the blood vessels are very close to the surface. The body uses this mechanism to eliminate blood for various reasons and in this comparative the nose and the uterus are very close. She looked me straight in the eye and said, "How close can they get?" Suddenly realising what she had said, thanked me very much for the explanation and changed the subject.

A patient attempted to explain some of the discomfort she was experiencing. She said, "Doctor my arms keep going to sleep at night and keeping me awake, do you think you can help?"

A woman explained that she was feeling the aches and pains of old age attacking her. I explained to her that old age generally doesn't hit with such immediate and acute pain, that it usually sneaks up on a person. She looked at me and said, "Do you think I'm suffering for the sins of my youth?"

A lesson of life: generally if we avoid eating what we eat most of, we will stay well.

A patient having trouble with her neck, explained that when she went to kiss her husband she couldn't bend her head back, and as a result had to kick him in the shins so that he'd bend over for her to kiss him. She then explained to me that before a family problem develops, she would like to get her neck fixed.

A patient with low back pain commented, "Doctor my back hurts like crazy. Do you think you can snap me out of it?"

A patient explained, "Doctor, I have this funny back and I thought I should come and see you before it gets bad. I'd much rather you see me at the funny stage than at the bad stage."

A patient attended the day after receiving treatment for a low back condition. I advised her to do light duties while her back was getting better. During the second visit she said to me, "Doctor, I have a question about the light duties that you recommended. My husband asked me to ask you how much weight must I lose to qualify for light duties?"

A patient attended with three young children, obviously a little distraught. She explained that her back was very painful. She said, "Doctor I think I have worked my back to the bone."

Chapter Fourteen

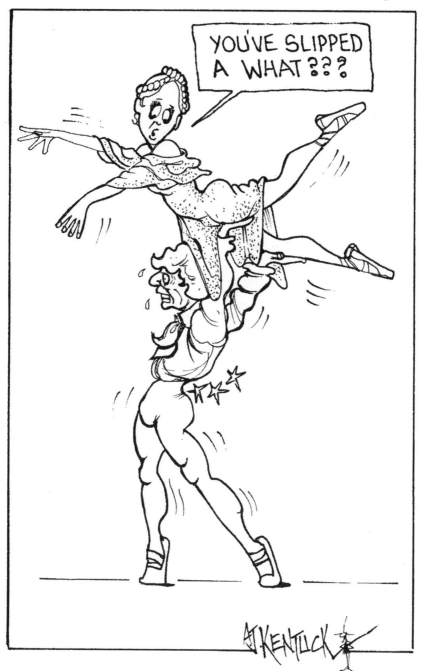

A patient explained that she had the day off work and took the opportunity to come and see me. I asked her if there was anything wrong that I should be aware of? She said, "Yes, I have Patricia-it is." I said, "Patricia-it is? I've never heard of that, what is it?" She said, "My boss's name is Patricia, she just kept rubbing me the wrong way and I didn't want to get too hot under the collar, so I took the day off work."

A democracy works well only when you have greed and corruption to finance it.

A patient was being treated for a low back problem. While positioning the patient, his back suddenly made a loud click. He looked up and smiled, saying, "Doctor, is this what you call premature manipulation?"

A patient explained that his back was extremely painful getting out of bed, but he couldn't determine whether it was his bed, pillow, back or wife. He said, "I want you to check out my back before I get into trouble make assumptions about the other factors."

Some things you always try to hide get bigger. For example, problems, weight, stomachs and lies.

Life speeds up with knowledge and slows down with ignorance. Awareness of opportunities makes life seem much faster.

Some people love being independent as long as they have a good partner to take care of them.

When man waters the garden he always misses something, but when God does it He usually gets everything.

A Patient arrived for consultation and explained, "Well doctor, today I don't think I have one good bone in my body."

Fear is man's attempt to justify his own ignorance.

A somewhat nervous patient said to me, "Doctor I don't know what to do, I get so tense when I relax; sometimes I think that my tension is all that's holding me together."

A patient was explaining how she had pain in her left leg, left arm and left shoulder. I asked her if there was anything else she could think of that was giving her trouble. She looked at me and said, "Yes, probably the leftovers."

Excitement and happiness in life are found in direct proportion to your ability to manage stress.

Woman receiving treatment for her back said, "Doctor, I'm not sure about the pains I am getting. Is it possible that I could be feeling a little nauseous after having an adjustment?" I said, "Well, that's possible." She said, "I thought I was pregnant." I said, "Well, I can't recall giving you an adjustment for that." She said that her tests were negative, but she was a little confused until she recalled that she couldn't remember having an adjustment for it at home either.

Expectant abuse: When one feels guilty about doing something someone else has asked of them.

Living a lie eventually makes you sick to death.

Dreams are what we live for; wishes are excuses for our fears.

A Patient explained that she was feeling every groan in her bones.

With enthusiasm and great gusto, a patient said, "Here I am Doctor, with your favourite joint."

The difficulty patients have in making their appointments is usually in direct proportion to how well they feel.

A patient was lamenting about finding help for her headaches and said, "Doctor you are my last hope, you're the cherry on top of the cake and you know what happens to the cherry if you can't do the job!"

The difference between work and slavery is love and purpose.

Chapter Fifteen

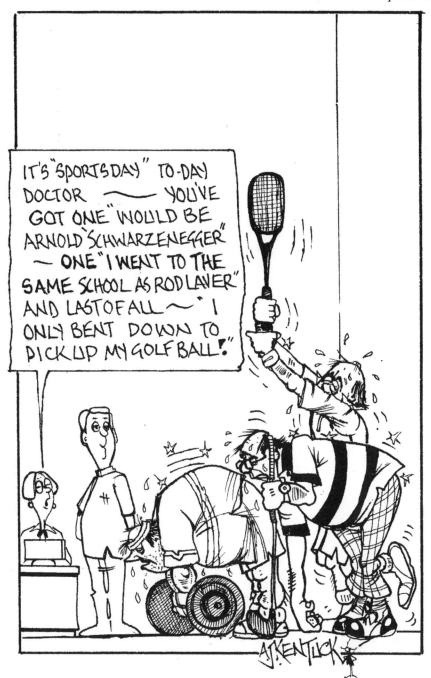

81

A patient complained about having pain when walking for extended distances and said, "Doctor I have trouble walking. I am walking with a trip and a skip, instead of a skip and a hop."

A patient explained, "Doctor I think I can feel my neck *coming on.* Do you think it could be a 'Four X [XXXX]' or a 'Tooheys' problem? Perhaps if I drank more beer I wouldn't feel the pain!"

After having his adjustment two days earlier a patient said, "Doctor, the morning after your adjustment I was unrecognisable." Thinking that I had caused some discomfort, I said, "Were you unrecognisable for the better or the worse?" Somewhat startled he said, "Definitely for the better."

During an examination I was dictating all the names of the patient's dysfunctional muscles to my assistant. The muscle names are Greek and Latin. At the end the older patient looked me straight in the eye and said, "You know doctor, this is just like being at church, you say all the same things that my priest does. I just know I'm going to feel better after you finish with me."

A female patient in her later 60's came in trying to describe the aches and pains that she felt. She said, "Doctor I think I am getting old and stiff. Do you think that's a difficult problem?" Before I could comment she continued, "I know it's not a difficult problem for a man my age, but for a woman it is different."

While adjusting a patient's low back she released a large amount of bowel gas. Not wanting to be embarrassed she looked me straight in the eye and said, "I'm so glad that I come to see you, you always get rid of all my bad farts." "Oops," she said, "I meant to say parts."

A patient was complaining about the intensity of discomfort she had and said, "Doctor be kind to me, if I was a horse you would take me out and shoot me." I said, "We'll have to do something else, I'm fresh out of bullets."

A patient somewhat anxious about the type of treatment she was going to receive, explained to me, "Doctor I missed you. It's been such a long time since I've been here I have nearly forgotten what pain was like."

Another patient trying hard to explain how she felt after her treatment said, "Doctor I had no idea how bad my pain was until it went."

A patient was explaining about the arthritis in his knees and how it was feeling better with treatment. He said to me, "For the first time in years my knees have felt good enough to let my wife sit on them, but now I've forgotten what to do next."

A patient was having problems organising an appointment. The receptionist said, "I think this time it should work out, we'll fit you in here." The patient responded, "Good I like to fit in where I am wanted most."

A patient was explaining how her daughter didn't like the mineral tablets that she had been prescribed. She said that they tasted like birdseed and asked her mother, "Do you think I'll look like a parrot when I finish them?"

After finishing work on a female patient to help reduce tension, she turned around and commented, "Oh Doctor, I feel like I have relapsed again. Oh I'm sorry, I mean relaxed!"

A patient obviously under some anxiety commented, "Doctor I feel like a nervous wreck and I think my family may be preparing to throw me overboard."

An overweight patient with an extremely sore low back said, "Doctor I think I have exceeded all my *limits* and I haven't even begun to lose weight." ["Limits" is a brand name for a weight-reducing biscuit.)

A patient trying desperately hard to describe to me how painful her headache was said, "My headache feels like a herd of elephants are dancing on top of my head and they aren't even light-weights."

Chapter Sixteen

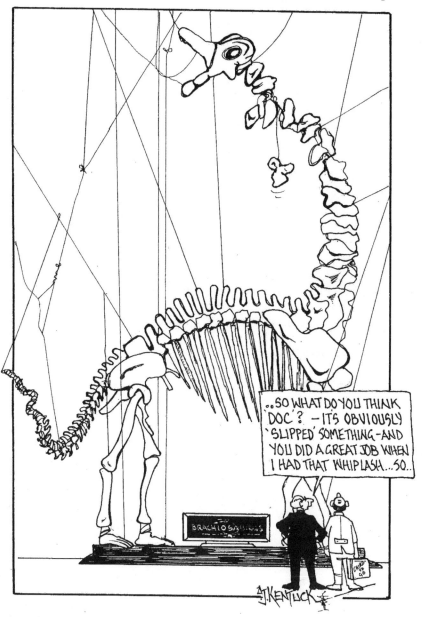

A patient trying to understand the change in posture she was experiencing said, "Doctor I feel like I am more forwards today and less backwards than I was yesterday, and I think it is all thanks to you fiddling around."

A patient somewhat at a loss to describe how she felt said, "Doctor I think I've got jiggered joints. What can you do with them?" How do you answer such a technical question?

A patient was enquiring about the function of my posturometer. He said to me, "What do you do with this?" I explained, "We use it to measure how crooked people are." He said, "In that case you'd better take it over to the Law Courts and after you finish with the magistrates, take it to Parliament House and see if you can help the politicians."

"Doctor I'd like to be in good shape for Christmas. Do you think you can make me into a nice present for somebody?"

"Doctor I think my problem is *twinges in my hinges*. Do you think you can fix them?'

A husband and wife attended my office. The wife was in obvious distress. Her husband tried to speak for her. He said, "Doctor I don't know what to do, my wife is a real pain!"

A patient explained during consultation: "Doctor I'm a real mess, I don't know where to start."

After treating a patient I asked how she felt. She straightened up and stretched then looked me straight in the eye and said, "I feel like I've been manhandled."

A patient was explaining to me some of the problems that blind people have. She said: There is a new pantyhose in Europe that has printed in Braille at the top of the thigh." I asked her what it said. She replied: "If you can read this, you have gone too far!"

A patient was reflecting on the number of visits she had had over the years and said to me, "Doctor you have no idea how much money I have saved in pharmacy bills since I have been coming to see you."

Another patient was trying to explain how much discomfort she was having in her legs and went on to comment, "My legs are giving me so much trouble I think I'll cut them off at my neck."

A patient said, "Doctor I have this terrible problem. I yawn all the time, I don't want to be known as a bore; do you think you can help?"

A patient was concerned about his height. He said, "Doctor do you think you can stretch me a few inches?" I responded, "I will do my best, but you will just have to be a little patient."

A patient explained: "Doctor I have a problem; when I think about you, I think about pain. Why is that?"

A little boy looking at my anatomical wall chart was reading the various names of the bones. He came to the pelvic area and said to me, pointing to the pubic region, "Doctor what is this *public arch?*"

A piano teacher explained that she had wrist problems and had difficulty with her practice. After I adjusted her wrists and fingers she said, "Doctor my fingers feel like they have stretched so far I'll probably be able to reach an extra octave."

"Doctor I never thought that there was a pain worse than having a baby – until I came here and you used some of those acupressure reflexes."

I was advising a patient, who was concerned about dieting, regarding the recommended nutritional supplement. After having her "taste test" the vitamin supplements, she said to me, "Doctor is this breakfast, lunch and dinner?" I said, "No, you have this *with* your breakfast, lunch and dinner."

Chapter Seventeen

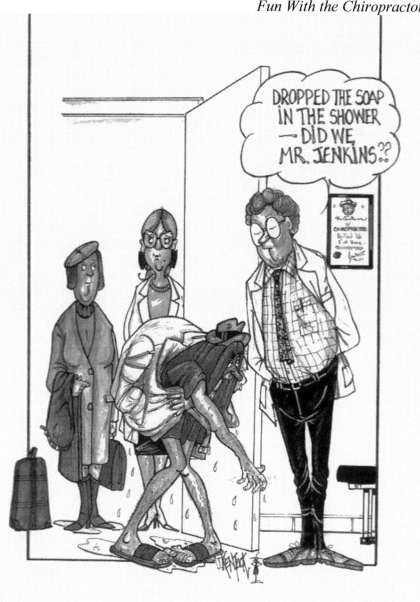

A patient explained that she would like a complete check-up in preparation for going away. She said, "Doctor I want you to give me every push and pull possible."

A patient was trying hard to describe the feelings she had with sciatic pain. She said, "Doctor I have this hot bum and hot legs, and don't know what to do with them."

A patient somewhat distressed while waiting for her appointment said: "Doctor, I have been a mass of pins and needles while I have been waiting for you, do you think this is why my husband says that I am as sharp as a tack?"

A patient explained the discomfort that she was feeling and said, "Doctor my arm feels like it's all screwed up and the strange thing is that I have a leg just like that too. What do you think you can do?"

A patient attended and as usual by way of introduction I asked him how he was feeling. He said, "I am aging with discretion. Trying not to make too much noise."

A patient explained that she had pain in her back that felt like toilet paper. I said, "Why do you say that?" She said, "Well the pain is just like toilet paper. It just keeps rolling on and on and on and on ..."

A patient attended who seemed much more relaxed than she had on her previous visit. I asked her how she was able to relax so much. She explained that she had joined a singles gourmet group. I asked her "What do you do?" She said, "We eat with each other!" After bursting out laughing she said, "No doctor, that's not all that we do, but we do enjoy each other's delights."

The only difference between love and hate is what you do to please your partner.

When it comes to knowledge, the brain can absorb no more than the seat can endure. When it comes to pain, the back can endure no more than the seat can feel.

A Patient exclaimed after her pressure point treatment: "Doctor, I didn't realise it was going to hurt so much. I feel like I have been to the Physio-terrorist."

A patient described the noises in her neck as she moved it. She said: "Doctor I feel just like a dog chewing its bone, the noise is incredible." I looked at her and said, "Well at least we didn't have to dig you up."

If you live long enough, you will die of old age.

A patient, the wife of a minister, explained after her adjustment: "Doctor, I didn't realise that the laying on of hands could be so beneficial. My husband performs laying on of hands in his work, but he doesn't do it nearly as firm as you do."

A patient was having some difficulty following my instructions during a muscle test of the fingers. She could not work out which fingers to put together for the test. She looked at me after some exasperation and said, "Doctor it is so hard doing these tests when I have so many choices."

A patient was complaining about how her back condition was affecting her marriage. She said to me that it was fortunate that marriage was such a give and take situation; in fact the most important part to her was to find a husband who could take all that she could give.

After treating a patient I said, "Your joints don't crack so much any more." He said: "Is that the same thing my wife means when she says I am not all I am cracked up to be?"

A patient commented on my greying hair. I said, "Each grey hair represents a new responsibility." She said, "Don't take it so seriously. All it means is that you are growing old *greys*fully."

A patient somewhat concerned about how to care for herself commented, "Doctor, should I do anything to avoid pain?" I answered, "Yes."

Chapter Eighteen

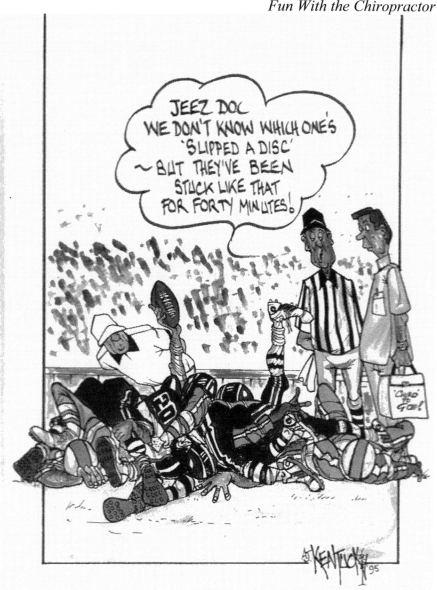

Donald McDowall

I was strapping a patient's strained elbow. When I explained how tight to make the strap, he asked, "Doctor do you mean it shouldn't be so tight that it is like a lamb's tail and falls off?"

A patient with a runny nose complained that he had "Dog's Disease". After I asked him why he called it "Dog's Disease", he said, "Only dogs deserve to have it."

Patient explained how she was having difficulty staying awake and at every opportunity would drop off to sleep. "You know, I think it's even possible that I could sleep on a clothes line."

A patient was feeling much better after her adjustment and explained to me. "Doctor, sometimes after you adjust me I feel like I am beside myself."

A patient attended with a cold. I asked her if she had received any advice about it. She said: "Yes, my medical doctor told me that if I fed it and took care of it for seven days it would go away, if I didn't it would take a week."

Do unto others as you would have others do unto you –
but don't expect others to do for you that which you have done
for them. Remember the golden rule is usually a one-way street.

Responsibility is what you feel when someone else
doesn't want to take it.

I never criticise age, because I keep catching up.

Control of your health depends upon your discipline.

Power is never given, but taken and used.

Why become a victim of everyone else's circumstances
when we have enough trouble being a victim of our own.

The human body is a very responsive mechanism. You
can pat it on the back and almost immediately it gets a swollen
head.

One of the gentlemen in my office had had a particularly
bad bout of flu and was still coughing a couple of weeks later.
One day he came in very excited, "I've been recommended a

natural remedy for my cough; it apparently works wonders on the flu – euthanasia!" *[Echinacea!]*

A patient complained of weak arms. He said, "My arms are so weak and painful, I can't even pick up a cup of tea." I asked, "What do you do?" She said, "I wait until it cools off and use a straw."

A patient had such a bad stiff neck that he couldn't even move it a fraction to the right. The left movement was okay, but movement to the right was completely locked. I asked, "How did you drive your car here with your neck like that, and not have an accident?" He replied: "Doc, I worked out if I only did left-hand turns I would get here without any trouble." His wife confirmed that he had circled all the left turn streets around my Clinic until he could park out the front.

A patient described the frustration she was experiencing with her back pain. Resolution of her insurance claim for her back injury was worrying her. She said, "Doctor I know what you do helps and I feel much better after my treatment, but every time I go to my lawyer and discuss the insurance claim, all my pain starts to come back." She told me that she explained this to her lawyer. I said: "What did he say?" She replied: "He said that

I would feel much better after I had a 'greenback' poultice for it."

Patient had an accident and hurt his back. He said that when playing on a trampoline with his children, he slipped and one of the children fell on him. I treated him and then asked him: "What do you think the lesson is in this experience?" He replied: "Don't let the kids on the trampoline, they just spoil your fun!"

Mrs. Bones was having a lot of trouble with her neck. I said, "What do you think causes this?" She said, "Sitting at a computer for long periods of time makes my neck very painful." I said, "Once I fix it for you, maybe you can get some recreation leave and give it a chance to get better." Somewhat frustrated she said: "Recreation leave? You mean 'wreck' leave!"

Chapter Nineteen

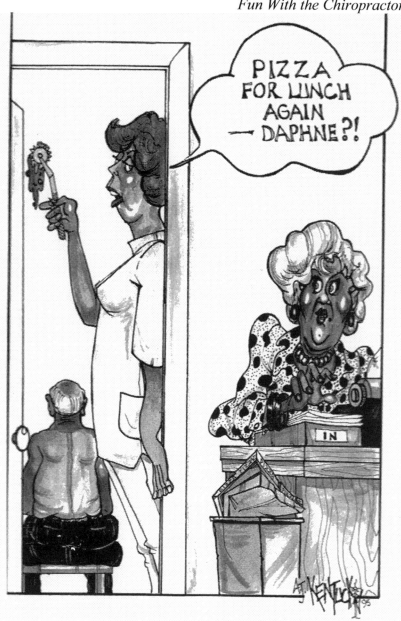

A secret to happiness is to find out what you feel good about and then do it.

Patient with a sore neck and shoulder pain explained that she had been babysitting her grandchildren. She felt perfectly fine before they arrived, but the problems seemed to develop after the afternoon babysitting. She said, "Doctor, do you think I could have been a victim of child abuse?"

Rewards are not a privilege. They are the result of performance.

After treating a patient with particularly noisy joints, he asked, "Doctor, do you think there's a good bone left in my body?"

While treating a family, the four-year-old daughter asked me, "Pop do you think I can go next?" "Why did you call me 'Pop'", I asked. Her mother replied, "When you explained last visit that the noises her joints made sounded like Rice Bubbles, she decided from then on to call you 'Pop'."

You have to understand the words you use, otherwise you only use the words you understand.

You get sick from doing what you don't like to do, or too much of what you do like to do.

Students are the teacher's teacher.

Your mind tells you the truth before you use your body. Your body tells you whether your mind was right after it is used.

Perception is always slanted. Gravity tells the truth.

Mr. Smith attended late in the day, obviously distressed, and said, "Doctor, everything feels like a mess. Do you think you could just erase me and start me all over again?"

A 70-year-old patient explained that he felt he was slowing down. I said, "What do you mean slowing down?" He answered, "Well, Doc, I'm getting a good day's work done, but it's taking me a week to do it."

A three-year-old came in with his mother to get his adjustment. He looked me in the eye and said, "I am here to have a massing-arch *[massage]*, but don't crack my neck."

Mrs Claus staggered into the clinic a few days before Christmas. I asked her what happened. She said she was suffering from: "shopping trolley shuffle that caused low back pain"!

Your body is only the vehicle. Where you are going in life is the real priority.

A patient, struggling to understand how to be patient with the chronicity of her problem said, "Doctor I think I am the longest-living terminal patient you have ever had."

I was giving a male patient instructions regarding care for his back. I told him he shouldn't do any vacuuming for at least a week. He said, "Doctor I don't know if the boss will approve of that. There is only democracy in our house as long as I do what I am told."

The constant quest for not keeping patients waiting was amusingly remedied by a doctor in England. He found the answer to stopping patient's complaints was to install a lotto gaming machine in his reception area. For every 15-minute interval he was late, the patient was eligible for a free turn. The receptionist noted that some patients would sit on the edge of their seats watching the clock, just hoping the doctor would be that extra few minutes late, so they could have a second turn. Here was a doctor who was not only an excellent diagnostician, but found the perfect remedy. One only wonders how many gambling addicts he created.

Feeling much better after her treatment, Mrs. Jones told me this joke her minister had told about a happy marriage in his sermon last Sunday: "A man, when marrying his new wife, didn't realise that her maiden name of "Miss Right" would, in reality, never change".

A patient so excited about the reduction of pain in her shoulder said, "My arm feels so much better I can actually lean on my elbow when I am having a cup of coffee."

If you don't think about what you do, you become a victim of your circumstances.

A patient attended complaining of lower leg cramps. After adjusting his feet, I suggested he do some exercise with them. He said, "The only exercise they get is when I put my foot in my mouth."

Donald McDowall

A patient came seeking a second opinion for a persistent problem. When I asked what was wrong, she said: "the previous doctor threw his hands in the air, said he didn't know and the only way to find the cause of this problem was with an autopsy!"

On his first visit to the Clinic Mr. Smith was describing his problem. He said, "Doctor my back is very sore. I feel like I have bones everywhere."

A mother was encouraging her 4 year old to come to the clinic and have his back checked after a fall off his bicycle. Much to the mother's amazement he shook his head and said: "I feel much better now, I don't need a thwacking *(cracking)* today!"

About the Author

Donald McDowall was born in Australia and is a practicing chiropractor in Canberra, Australia. He has conducted a private practice since graduation from Palmer College of Chiropractic (Iowa, USA) in 1974. He is a Diplomate of the National Board of Chiropractic Examiners and a Member of the International Board of Applied Kinesiology since 1978. He has continually served in leadership positions of his profession as well as community organisations.

Dr McDowall has authored numerous papers in professional journals. He has also published four books: *A Clinical Approach to Health Through Food Programming* (1976), *Psychic Surgery – The Philippines Experience* (1993), *Healing – Doorway to the Spiritual World* (1998) and *Clinical Pearls for Better Health* (2002). In 1998 he developed a peer-reviewed, award-winning web site of information about chiropractic and healing (http://www.chiroclinic.com.au/pubs).

Dr McDowall's interest in the subtleties of healing has caused him to explore and gather information from many parts of the world. He has lectured in the United States, Europe, New Zealand and Australia.

Dr McDowall and his wife, Annie, have nine children.

Made in the USA
Lexington, KY
04 April 2010